Register This Book and Get Free Updates and Free Videos

To get free updates to this book and access to videos that will show you how to utilize strategies in this book and an invitation to online interactive livecasts to meet the author & ask questions, visit www.TheBenefitsOfSmokingBonus.com or text BOS to 58885 or text your name and email address to (609) 455-1224 Or scan this QR code:

The

Benefits

of

Smoking

Why It's So Hard to Quit Smoking &
What You Can Do About It!

Carol L Rickard, LCSW, TTS

Well YOUniversity® Publications

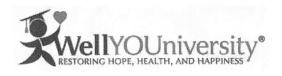

The Benefits of Smoking
Why It's So Hard to Quit Smoking & What You Can Do About It!

Carol L Rickard, LCSW, TTS

Published by:
Well YOUniversity® Publications,
A Division of WellYOUniversity, LLC
888 LIFETOOLS

The author & publisher of this book do not dispense medical advice nor prescribe the use of this material as a form of treatment.

Disclaimer: The purpose of this material is educational only. Please see you doctor before starting any health program or concerning any medical advice you may need.

ISBN-13: 978-09821010-8-7

Table of Contents

Foreword

No

This is not a book about **encouraging** people to smoke! However, the title honestly represents my personal belief *there are* benefits to smoking. And if these benefits are not addressed specifically, it is nearly impossible for a person to **sustain** their success with quitting tobacco.

The three benefits are as follows:

1) Preventing a person from experiencing withdrawal symptoms.

2) Helping a person cope with their stress & emotions.

3) Becoming a person's '*always there for you*' friend.

This is **NOT** A Quit Plan!

It's a *TOOLBOX!* My aim is to give you all the tools you need to be successful!

Introduction

If YOU are someone who's tried to
in the past *without success* or
someone who's been considering quitting
then you are in the

right place at the right time!

For over **22** years, I've been helping people in
hospital based programs successfully change
their **health habits**. There is *no more important*
habit to change than to quit smoking.

I believe people are already smart enough
when it comes to being healthy.

You **KNOW WHAT TO DO!**

It's the '*DOING*' or *lack of it* that

keeps you stuck where you are.

I can help *change* that!

I doubt you have read a 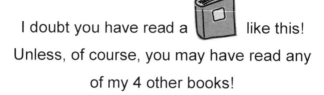 like this!
Unless, of course, you may have read any
of my 4 other books!

Along with **simple** easy to understand chapters,
I tend to use a lot of pictures, analogies,
& word art to make the information stick in the brain!

Here at WellYOUniversity® I describe our
approach as "Whole Brain Wellness".
It's what makes our services & resources
different from all others!

KNOWLEDGE is the left brain at work.
This is where YOU *know* what to do!

Because we use "pictures" and "images"
as our foundations, we end up
tapping in to the other side of the brain –

the right side!

So both sides of a brain are focused on the same thing! The end result is getting people to

put knowledge in to ACTION!

Whole Brain Wellness was developed as a result of working in treatment settings where patient's concentration & memory were limited.

Over the years, our approach has enabled us to help a great many people have success with **changing around their health habits!**

You see, I've had the idea for this book in my head for *many* years.

It wasn't *until* I had the right training about tobacco dependence that it could come to life!.

In 2011, I completed UMDNJ's Tobacco Dependence Treatment Specialist training. It is one of **only 11** ATTUD *accredited* programs in the country.

Having utilized this training in my work at the **HOSPITAL** H over the past 3 years –

I'm confident in putting this book out to you!

At first glance, you might think this book was actually promoting smoking! Upon a closer look, you'll see that **it does no such thing!**

Rather, it calls attention to WHY it's so hard to quit & offers you the "tools" to be successful.

Finally, you can quit! Or as I like to say:

Kick Cigarettes Butts!

You will find this book divided in to two parts:

Part 1 is designed to help you understand

WHY

it's so hard to quit smoking.

It's not your fault!

Biology plays the most critical role
and the physical piece cannot be ignored.

Here you will learn about the "*tools*" available
that can help you manage this **physical piece.**

Part 2 is designed to help you understand

WHAT

you can do to *ensure* your success.

If you don't take care of the '*behavioral*' piece –
any success will be **short lived**.

I've always believed that you

Can't just *give up* cigarettes,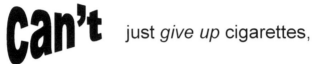

which have become most smokers
main coping tool,

without **replacing** them with other
healthy coping tools!

My promise to you:

By the time you have finished this book,
you'll have all you need to be successful &
finally Kick Cigarettes Butts!

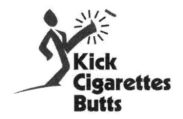

**Kick
Cigarettes
Butts**

SM 2014 Well YOUniversity, LLC

My Story

As you *read* through this book,
you will *learn more about me* and
the impact smoking has had in my life.

.

I come from a family of smokers.

Most of those who smoked & kept smoking
were dead by the age of **62**

Little did I know that God would put me on a path
to have a DIFFERENT OUTCOME for myself
& to *help so many others get on a different path.*

I am **grateful** for my life experiences & lessons,
as they have been the gifts I use to help and teach
others how to **live well TODAY!**

I feel *privileged* to be able to write this book and offer
these tools to BENEFIT so many others.

My first memories of cigarettes are the times I would be sitting in the back seat of our station wagon.

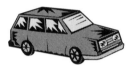

I was just 6 or 7 & we had a five hour drive from our home in Burbank up to our campsite at **Ducey's Lodge** located in Bass Lake, California.

My brother would be *on one side of the car* and I *on the other*, our **windows cracked open** just a little because the dual zone air conditioning was running and we didn't want to get in **trouble!**

We sat with our HEADS TILTED UP so that our mouths were positioned right at the opening of the window so that we could get a

BREATH OF FRESH AIR!

My *last memories* of smoking involve my mother:

Gloria R. Rickard

I actually wished a book like this had been

available when she was still alive.

My mother's dependence on cigarettes was

so powerful

that despite her **many health issues** she still kept

smoking right up until her death on August 23, 1989

My mother's story goes like this:

Severe asthma and *kept SMOKING*....

Several heart attacks and *kept SMOKING*....

Quadruple bypass surgery and *kept SMOKING*....

Cardiac arrest hours after bypass & *kept SMOKING*

A hole in her chest, where staples would have been. They

busted during CPR & it was too risky to redo them

AND *SHE KEPT SMOKING*........

I had **no idea** what she was *up against* when I kept begging her to QUIT to save her life.

I don't think she did either.

I now realize she didn't stand much of a chance trying to quit on her own.

I wish I'd know then WHAT I KNOW NOW….,.

My hope is it's not too late for **you to learn NOW!**

~ To Living Well TODAY! ~

Carol

Our Starting Point

You can either circle your answers below or on a separate piece of paper. Don't skip this part!

T = True   F = False

1) Cancer is caused by the nicotine in cigarettes. T   F

2) You can't smoke while wearing a patch. T   F

3) Half of all smokers will die from a tobacco related disease. T   F

4) Natural tobacco is safe to smoke. T   F

5) E Cigarettes are a safe alternative to real ones. T   F

6) 70% of all lung cancer is tobacco caused. T   F

7) There are 45 carcinogens found in cigarette smoke. T   F

8) It's okay to use a nicotine patch at the *same time* as using nicotine gum or lozenge . T F

9) Quitting cold turkey is the least effective approach. T F

10) When smokers take a puff from a cigarette, it takes about 30 seconds for the nicotine to reach the reward center in the brain. T F

We will come back to these questions a little later!

Part 1

WHY It's So Hard To Quit

Register This Book and Get Free Updates and Free Videos

To get free updates to this book and access to videos that will show you how to utilize strategies in this book and an invitation to online interactive livecasts to meet the author & ask questions, visit www.TheBenefitsOfSmokingBonus.com or text BOS to 58885 or text your name and email address to (609) 455-1224 Or scan this QR code:

Up In Smoke!

Up In Smoke

Before we go on, I have a **?** I'd like to ask:

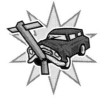

How would you feel about going to work *every day*

in a car that has a 50% chance of

getting in an accident & you dying?

Would you - Keep using that car?

or

STOP using it?

Well, if you are like most of the people I have asked,

You'd STOP using that car!

Those odds aren't so good!

Did you know that a smoker faces those same odds?

50% of ALL SMOKERS

will die from *tobacco related disease*.

That is the same as if YOU were driving

THAT CAR to work every day!

Now, I don't write that to *scare* anyone in to quitting!

The truth is, I think enough people **already know** that smoking is really BAD for their health.

Sometimes, our brains can filter out information that hits *too close to home*.
It's a little harder to filter out images!

However, I myself was surprised when I learned in my

TTS training that **90%** of

ALL lung cancers are tobacco caused.

Smoking is also the leading cause of **COPD**, which is a disease that over time impairs your ability to breath.

In the U.S., **COPD** includes 2 main conditions:

Emphysema

&

Chronic Bronchitis

My mother had also developed emphysema.
It got so bad, she could only walk short distances.

You can't get rid of **COPD** once you have it. There is no cure….only ways to slow down its progression.

Many people have it AND don't even know it.

I saw it '*suck the life*' right out of my mother.

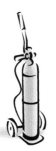

She had to have a little oxygen tank she carried around with her everywhere she went.

An exercise I'd like you to try –

Only if your health *allows* you to do it!

Hold a coffee stirring straw in your mouth, pinch your nose closed, & breath in & out through that straw!

Now, jog or walk fast in place for 30 seconds!

That's what it's like to have COPD.

It's The Smoke That Kills!

When I attended my TTS Training, one of the first

things I was surprised to learn was that

nicotine DID NOT cause cancer.

All my life, I thought it was the **nicotine**

that was *so bad for a person's health.*

Wow! That one was a stunner!

So if nicotine doesn't cause cancer – **WHAT DOES?**

The answer lies in the bucket below!

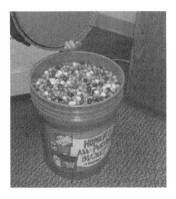

How many peanut M & M's

do you think there are in this 5 gallon bucket?

There are a **GRAND TOTAL of 7,000!**

(And YES, I counted *every single one* of them!!)

It just so happens that this is the

same number of compounds found in

CIGARETTE SMOKE.

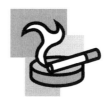

These **7,000** compounds include the following:

ACETONE - found in *nail polish remover*

ARSENIC - found in good old *rat poison*

AMONIA -   found in *cleaning products*

SULFURIC ACID – found in *car batteries*

BUTANE – found in *cigarette lighters*

FORMALDEHYDE – found in *funeral homes*

Also included in these **7,000 compounds are**

65 known carcinogens.

It's *these compounds* that are causing
cancer and a host of other diseases.

Something I'd like to point out here:
This is in **SMOKE** ONLY,

not *the cigarettes themselves.*

When I learned this I was astounded. For the first time,
I understood the **dangers of second hand smoke** –

A person *doesn't* have to **be the one**
smoking the cigarette in order to be exposed
to all those different compounds.

Just *breathing* in the smoke does it.

Okay,
I know someone, somewhere
is reading this right now &
thinking to themselves:

"Yea, I believe it about those *big tobacco* cigarettes. It's all the stuff they put in them!"

"But my **natural tobacco cigarettes** are *safe to smoke.* They don't have those chemicals or additives."

That is exactly *what I thought too!* I always believed my sister's 'natural tobacco' cigarettes were healthier!

I WAS WRONG!!!!

While it's true they may not have additives,

there are **2** important points to understand:

1) Many of the unhealthy compounds come from the act of 'burning' itself –

natural stuff or **not**!

2) The tobacco plant itself

contains sources of unhealthy compounds.

This is **why** other forms of tobacco are also

known to cause **cancer & disease**.

It is important to understand

there is **no such thing**

as

safe tobacco.

Whether it's:

smoked

snuffed

chewed

or snussed!

It's ALL in Your Head!

Nicotine

As I mentioned earlier,

I had *always thought* it was the **nicotine** in cigarettes

that was so damaging to health.

What I came to understand is that nicotine can be

VERY DANGEROUS

in another way…..

It has power over our brains similar
to that of other addictive drugs -
including heroin and cocaine.

Nicotine activates the same reward pathways

as these other drugs, increasing levels

of **dopamine** in our brain.

Dopamine

is a key **feel good chemical** in our brains!

What makes nicotine even **more dangerous**

is that *inhalation*

is the *FASTEST* route to the brain.

It only takes **10 seconds**

from when a person takes a puff of a cigarette

for the nicotine to reach the reward center in the brain!

10 Seconds!!

Nicotine is an addiction –

not a habit people choose.

Science can now show us how once the brain **becomes**

dependent on nicotine, it *screams* for more!

And the body begins to go through

withdrawal *when* it doesn't get it.

You've probably experienced or witnessed this before!

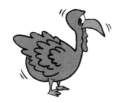

Have you tried to *quit* before

trying to go '**cold turkey**'?

If not, ever had a friend, coworker, or family member

who has tried to quit smoking by going '**cold turkey**'?

How would you describe how you or that person acted?

Bubbly, cheerful, delightful & fun to be around.

or

Irritable, angry, nasty, & NO fun to be around.

I have run the other direction from coworkers

I knew who were trying to !

There are **several symptoms** people experience when going through nicotine withdrawal:

Depressed Mood

Insomnia

Irritability

Frustration

Anger

Anxiety

Difficulty concentrating

Restlessness

Increased appetite

Weight gain

Most importantly is the fact these symptoms

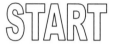

within a few hours of the last smoke!

This leads us to……

Benefit #1 of smoking

It keeps YOU from *experiencing*

WITHDRAWAL!

There *is a much safer way* to avoid withdrawal
& we'll get to this next.

For now, it is important to understand how you
may try to avoid these symptoms – which usually
means lighting up another cigarette!

The Replacements!

Keys to Success

Here are some *pretty amazing* statistics!

Out of all the U.S. adult cigarette smokers:

* Approx. **68%** report they *WANT* to quit completely.

* Approx. **44%** report they *TRY TO QUIT* each year.

My 1st thought is: **Good for you!**

My 2nd thought is: *How sad....*

Sad because only a very small percentage of those smokers may succeed the 1st time & then could give up..

Trying to quit on your own is *the toughest road* to go down - **ONLY 4-7%** of smokers quit for good this way.

However, THERE IS HOPE!!!!

First:

Tobacco use & dependence

is now viewed as a *chronic disease.*

This recognizes smokers will typically **cycle through**
periods of remission & relapse
on their way to freedom from tobacco.

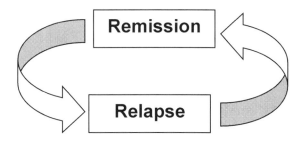

Second:

Current treatment approaches have been
shown to be much more effective than in the past.

By the time you finish this chapter,
I promise a new road to quitting will emerge before you!

One that works!

NRT – What Is It?

Hopefully you are getting a *clearer understanding* of just how **powerfully addictive** smoking can be.

This brings me to the focus of this section:

Nicotine Replacement Therapy or NRT

NRT products were introduced **30** *years ago* to help people stop smoking.

Nicotine gum & patches

were originally approved through **FDA** new drug process between 1984 and 1992.
They were *only available by prescription.*

NRT was shown to be safe & effective in

helping people stop smoking.

The key was supplying controlled amounts of nicotine to *ease the withdrawal* symptoms during quitting.

NRT gum & patches were switched to

over-the-counter (OTC) status

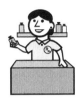

between 1996 & 2002.

Research had shown they were safe for use
without prescription.

The nicotine lozenge & mini lozenge were approved

directly for OTC use in *2002 & 2009*.

There are **2** other NRT products:

nicotine inhalers & nasal spray.

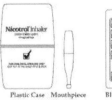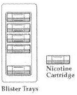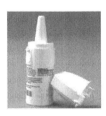

However, both require a prescription.

The Surest Way to Fail!

The one sure way to FAIL fast

is **NOT** *use enough* **NRT!**

There are several considerations when it comes to determining HOW MUCH NICOTINE you need.

These include:

How much *time until your 1st smoke in the am?*

How *many cigarettes do you smoke a day?*

Do you *re-light & if so, how many x's in a day?*

It is important to get some *guidance* on this.

Quit lines & networks will vary state by state.

A few good places to help **identify resources:**
Your State Quit Center / Line
The American Lung Association
A local hospital / medical center
The American Cancer Society

FDA Approved

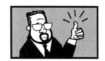

There are actually a total of **7** FDA **approved**

smoking *cessation aides* for you to be aware of.

We talked about NRT in the last section.
This included the 3 OTC's
as well as *2 others* by **prescription only**.

The 2 other FDA approved smoking

cessation aides contain <u>no</u> <u>nicotine</u> at all.

They work a *little differently*.

They are the prescription medications:

buproprion SR (Zyban®)

and

varenicline tartrate (Chantix®).

You may have already heard of them

or seen ads....

They BOTH work, in different ways,

on the receptors in the brain that

are *involved with nicotine dependence.*

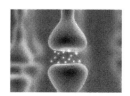

I like to think these 2 medications as

working on our brain from the ***inside-out***

while NRT does its work from the ***outside-in***!

It is STRONGLY RECOMMEND

that before starting

ANY type of smoking cessation program,

you *discuss it with your healthcare provider.*

Together you'll be able to determine

which may *serve your health needs*

best.

Evidence Based Practice

Today, there are

1,000's

of studies & trials involving the use and safety of NRT.

It has been shown to be an

evidence based practice

in the treatment of *tobacco dependence*.

Other studies have also shown that *counseling*
in a **variety of forms** is *effective*
for helping smokers quit.

This counseling can take many different forms such as:

➢ A 3-5 minute conversation with a healthcare provider.

➢ Joining a support group (a Quit Group) live or online.

➢ Reaching out to telephone counseling which should be
available through your state's quit line.

> Setting a Quit Date & having a plan around it.

In addition:

There is a good deal of research showing us

that the combination of interventions works even better!

Counseling & NRT together is more effective

& gives people the **greatest levels of success**.

NRT medications *can also* be effectively combined

to further reduce the likelihood of

Withdrawal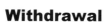

Relapse

Patch + Gum or lozenge = ↑success

Myths Exposed

#1 – *"Won't I just get 'addicted' to this nicotine like I did the cigarettes?"*

The speed of nicotine reaching the brain via smoking is one of the reasons you get so dependent on cigarettes.

 So much so,

I have heard *smoking* be referred to as the 'crack' of nicotine.

This is what makes smoking one of the

most difficult

dependencies to deal with.

While there *is* a possibility a person

may become dependent on the

nicotine in replacement therapy –

First and foremost,

it is **NOT** one of the **65 carcinogens!**

Secondly,

it does **NOT** contain the other

6999 compounds you take in

when smoking a cigarette!

IMPORTANT!!!

 can have an effect on

some medications....

Speak with your healthcare provider

before starting any type of quit effort.

If they *aren't knowledgeable* than contact your states

Quit Line or American Lung Association

for a referral to someone who is!

#2 – *"I tried those patches before –*
They didn't work.
All I wanted to do was go smoke!"

I've heard people say this about **ALL** the different

over-the-counter NRT products.

What I say back to them is:

The reason the patch

(or which other NRT product it is)

isn't working is *probably* because

you are not getting enough nicotine

to **replace** what you were smoking!!!

Many times, people need to *either* -

use more of the NRT they're using

or

combine it with **another** NRT product.

This can be hard to figure out on your own.

41

It's *also a reason why* it can be **so beneficial**

for you to talk to a Quit Line or Quit Center

counselor who has the training to help figure it out!

What is **SAD** to me is

YOU *trying to figure things out on you own*

& when they don't work,

you will most likely give up & **stop trying**.....

Getting back in *that car* with

the **50%** chance *you will die*.

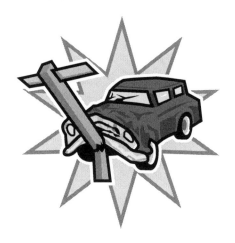

#3 – *"If you smoke while wearing a patch, you could have a heart attack."*

 If you look at an old box of patches, you will find the **warning** in the directions to *not smoke while wearing a patch.*

While this once was thought to be the case, **it no longer is!**

In fact, the FDA is in the process of making **new label changes** on NRT products!

This includes removing the warnings:

➢ Do not use an NRT if you're still smoking.

➢ Do not use with another NRT

This comes after the FDA reviewed scientific research on the safety of NRT

&

determined *the warnings & limitations* on the directions

were no longer necessary.

** Again**

If you find yourself smoking

AND

Using the patch,

It's a *pretty good sign* that you may need to kick up

the **strength** of the patch or add in another NRT.

A very common combination is

the patch & the lozenge or gum!

#4 – *"My e-cigarette doesn't put out any smoke so it's healthier, right?"*

I know it's a pretty safe bet I'll hear this one!

So, let's talk a little bit about *electronic cigarettes* or as they are otherwise called, e-cigarettes.

When I was at a recent tobacco treatment training for mental health settings, there were *a lot of questions* about electronic cigarettes!

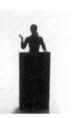

Here are a few key points:

Point #1

There is NO manufacturing oversight or regulation.

(at least at the time this edition is being written)

This means that **NOBODY** *knows* **WHAT** *is being put in them!*

*** As noted on the FDA's website,

One sample tested was found to contain

diethylene glycol

a toxic chemical used in antifreeze.

A word of caution I'd like to note:

We went down this same road

with tobacco cigarettes *many decades* ago

& looked where we landed!

Can we really afford to make the same mistake?

Point #2

Many products are coming from outside the US.

Can you really **TRUST** you're getting

a **SAFE** product?

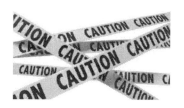

Point #3

There is no evidenced-based research
at this time demonstrating e cigarettes
are effective at helping people quit smoking.

However, I have *heard* *from some people* who **SAY**

it's been their e-cig that's gotten them to

stop smoking!

I still wonder if they've just changed poisons?!

Point #4

Electronic cigarettes exist **without many** of the

SAFEGUARDS *built in to real cigarettes* to protect

young people from becoming addicted to nicotine.

The concern is this could then

take away from the progress made

smoking rates **amongst young people.**

In closing out this topic,

I'd just like to say, I believe

e-cigarette users should become

EDUCATED about their brands.

Question:

WHERE are they made?

HOW are they made?

&

HOLD companies accountable for

truth and disclosure.

E Cigarettes still have a ways to go

before you can truly say they're SAFE.

my best advice **is BUYER BEWARE!**

Our Starting Point – Revisited!

You can either circle your answers below or on a separate piece of paper. What did you learn!

T = True   F = False

1) Cancer is caused by the nicotine in cigarettes. T F

2) You can't smoke while wearing a patch. T   F

3) Half of all smokers will die from a tobacco related disease. T F

4) Natural tobacco is safe to smoke. T   F

5) E Cigarettes are a safe alternative to real ones. T F

6) 70% of all lung cancer is tobacco caused. T   F

7) There are 45 carcinogens found in cigarette smoke. T F

8) It's okay to use a nicotine patch at the same time as either the nicotine gum or lozenge . T F

9) Quitting cold turkey is the least effective approach. T F

10) When smokers take a puff from a cigarette, it takes about 30 seconds for the nicotine to reach the reward center in the brain. T F

I am willing to bet you did pretty well on this one!

See the key at the end of the book if needed!

Part 2

What You Can Do About It!
How to manage life without tobacco!

Register This Book and Get Free Updates and Free Videos

To get free updates to this book and access to videos that will show you how to utilize strategies in this book and an invitation to online interactive livecasts to meet the author & ask questions, visit www.TheBenefitsOfSmokingBonus.com or text BOS to 58885 or text your name and email address to (609) 455-1224 Or scan this QR code:

Got Tools?

Do you have a tool box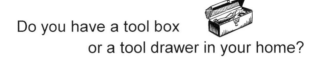
        or a tool drawer in your home?

I'll bet money you have either **one or the other!**

Just as we have tools around to take care
of the 'physical' problems in our life,
we also need to have tools around to take care
of the 'emotional' problems in our life..

Now, I have another question for you!

        Have you ever taken a knife and
        tried to use it as a screwdriver?

Be honest!

(Usually when I ask this question in my workshops,
EVERYONE in the room raises their hands!)

How did it work?
                Not *too* well, right?

At some point, we have to come back with
a real screwdriver and fix it again!

Now, just in case you are one of those people
who thinks the 'knife' worked just fine –

This question is for you!

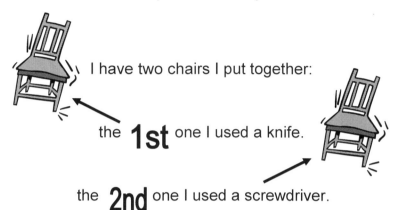

I have two chairs I put together:

the **1st** one I used a knife.

the **2nd** one I used a screwdriver.

Which chair do you want to sit in?!

I *thought so*..... the *screwdriver* chair!

Let's face it –

having the **'right tool'** for a job

can make all the difference

between **success** & failure.

I don't know about you....

I want to only have to do the job ONCE !

Survival Tools vs. LifeTools

  I believe the same kind of situation can happen when we are faced with 'emotional' problems.

We just grab at something quickly to help us deal with a situation,

I call these **Survival Tools.**

These are all the things we may have used to help us get through the tough times in life.

To help us **SURVIVE** ....

And in many instances,

they do help us – temporarily.

The problem is that many of these

SURVIVAL TOOLS

go on to *become* the problem.

Let me share a couple of examples:

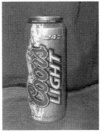

Coors Light is a registered
trademark of Coors Brewing Co.

What you are looking at is a picture of one of my old
SURVIVAL TOOLS.

It was December of 1976 when I overheard a
conversation *I wasn't suppose to*. I learned my father
was dying from cancer. I was 14 at the time,
just in my freshman year at Yosemite High School.

Now, I didn't tell anyone what I had heard…

Instead, I started stealing liquor from my parents.
We had just sold a bar & restaurant so there was
PLENTY of alcohol for me to get my hands on.

Also, my parents were busy dealing with my father so
no one noticed if anything was missing.

The truth be told, if my family had known how much I'd
been drinking – I know I would have been put in rehab.

Luckily for me, drinking

did not stay my survival tool.

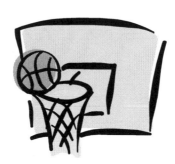

Became my **LIFETOOL!**

You could find me on a court somewhere

shooting for hours on end

&

the drinking came to a stop.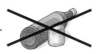

Unfortunately, in May of 1977,

I had a new **SURVIVAL TOOL** emerge –

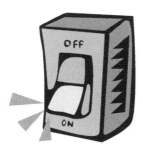

It was 6:00 o'clock in the morning on May 2, 1977.
I had just woken up & was on my way down the hallway
to get ready for school when my Mom stopped me.

As she told me I wouldn't be going to school today
because *my father had just passed away*, I remember
wrapping my arms around her and saying "It'll be okay."

My world instantly changed........

In that moment, which I can recall as if it were
yesterday, I also remember making
<u>a very conscious decision -</u>

*I would just go on with my life as if my father had
never been there to begin with…..*

I flipped my emotions switch

OFF.

It stayed my **SURVIVAL TOOL** for a very long time

It wasn't until my early **30**'s that I realized what had once helped me **SURVIVE** was now interfering with my life and preventing me from **LIVING**.

It started to interfere with a *very important relationship*.

I had a choice: keep on not dealing with my emotions in a very healthy way or change and learn a new way

 I didn't want to lose the relationship, so I started seeing a therapist for counseling.

I think of counseling as sort of a way to

learn more about yourself.

We don't know what we don't know!

Sometimes we need help from an objective party, outside our family and friends, to help guide us in the discovery to learn more about ourselves.

(I didn't realize the connection between my relationship problems & the emotion switch until I was in therapy!)

What I came to learn is:

Emotions are just like coins –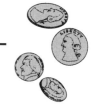

There are

2 sides to them & they can't be

separated!

In order to FEEL joy, love, happiness….

we must also feel sadness, anger, & pain

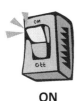
With my emotion switch back on

life has become much richer!!

ON

NOTE: If you can find yourself relating to my story,

and realize you "disconnect" from your feelings,

it may be important for you seek out professional help

to assist you in sorting through the issues & emotions.

There is one more example of **SURVIVALTOOLS**

I want to talk about –

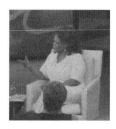

We all know who this is!

It is no secret that Oprah struggled

with her weight for many years…

I remember seeing her, in 1988, come out on her show

wearing those really skinny jeans,

pulling a wagon behind her

which represented all the weight she lost.

The success lasted only a short time!

It took her many more years to figure out **the secret:**

she used food as a way of coping with emotions!

I hope by now you begin to have a clearer picture of

what **SURVIVAL TOOLS** are &

why we need to swap them out for **LIFETOOLS!**

Could Smoking be your SURVIVALTOOL?

BENEFIT #2 – Your primary coping tool!

Keys to Changing
Your Tools!

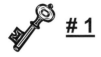 **# 1**

YOU are the one who must decide....

If what you're doing in life is working or not?

No one can answer this for you!

The fact remains that no matter what someone else

tells us or how hard they try to get us to change....

We must make the decision ourselves!

Otherwise,
change will be very short-lived
if it happens at all!

Steven Covey says it best:

"The gate of CHANGE
can only be opened from the inside"

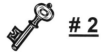 <u>**# 2**</u>

It is important not to *invalidate* the old tools….

I think it is very important **not** to beat yourself up over past behaviors. It doesn't matter if your old tools have been smoking, food, alcohol, work, or anything else

I think it is also very important to validate the fact these old **SURVIVAL TOOLS** *helped us do just that:* **SURVIVE**

I am where I am today because those early **SURVIVAL TOOLS** were a part of my life. Instead of looking at them with guilt & shame, I see them for what they were: some things I *'grabbed at'* to help me get through the **VERY difficult times in my life**

Simply put – they are tools that I no longer choose because I have healthier ones I can use!

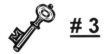 **# 3**

YOU are the only one….

One of my mentor's, the late Jim Rohn has a great line:

"You can't pay somebody else
to do your push-ups for you!"

I hate to break the news to you –

<u>We</u> are the only ones that can make these changes!

In order to be successful,

We must take **100%** responsibility!

&

We must **DO**

what we **DON"T FEEL LIKE DOING!**

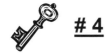 **# 4**

Watch out for the COMFORT ZONES!!

One of the greatest challenges of change

is that we are

comfortable with what we know.

We must be on the look out & notice when

we are going back to our old 'comfort zones".

Trust me, **this WILL happen**!

The key is to be on the look out for it,

recognize it is happening, and

then take action to get ourselves back on track!

I love the exercise we do in my workshops that helps

people to experience this for themselves. I learned it in

a training from Jack Canfield, one of the authors of the

"Chicken Soup for The Soul" series.

Here's how it goes!

Put your hands together in front of you, interlocking your fingers. (like the picture!)
Use left elbow to hold the book open!!

Now, leave everything the way it is but reverse the thumbs so they are the opposite of what they were!

Go ahead and do it now!

How does it feel?

At first, it will feel kind of uncomfortable!

You may be *tempted* to go right back to the other way, which feels <u>more</u> <u>comfortable</u>.

Go ahead & resist the urge & hold them in this position!
You will notice it starts to feel a little less weird!
Hold it even longer and it will actually

start to feel more comfortable.

This is a great way to reinforce what happens to us when we try to make changes in our lives.

It FEELS UNCOMFORTABLE!

We have to keep practicing the new behavior so we start to establish a new comfort zone!

Besides the natural tendency to want to stay in our comfort zones, there's one other HUGE stumbling block to making change:

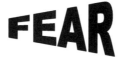

It is said we are born with **TWO** fears:

1) the fear of falling

2) the fear of loud noises

and all the others we learn!

What fears have you learned that you'd like to get rid if?

The next chapter will give you some tools for the job!

Get Moving!

Breaking Through Fear

There are several tools I teach to help my patients bust through fear & make healthy changes in their lives. I would like to share them with you! (These are the very same tools I live by!)

"Words can be powerful, put in to action, they become life changing!"

Carol L Rickard

Tool # 1

If you always do
what you've always done,

You'll always get
what you've always gotten,

Because if nothing changes....

NOTHING CHANGES!

Author Unknown

(I think this kind of speaks for itself!)

<u>Tool # 2</u>

One of the best books I ever read

&

the one that helped me really learn to
manage my fears:

"Who Moved My Cheese"
by Dr. Spencer Johnson.

If you haven't read this, I strongly recommend it!

It is a short story, about 90 pages long,
about these little characters who live in a maze
and are forced to deal with change.

It can be a LIFE CHANGER.....

You'll have to look for the book in
the *business sections.*

However,

it truly is more of a **Life Lesson's** story!

Tool # 3

It was during the first time I played an audio version of **"Who Moved my Cheese"** for my patients when I came up with this next tool.

I was sitting there, thinking about how to help people **see** change in a different way so they would welcome & embrace it rather than be afraid of it. I came up with:

Creating

Healthy

And

New

Growth

Experiences

2014 COPYRIGHT Well YOUniversity Publications
Taken from "Words At Work"
Licensed by Well YOUniversity, LLC

73

Tool # 4

While we don't get to control the events in our lives,

We *do get to control* <u>our</u> <u>response</u> to them!

We either **make our choice**

or **let fear** make it for us!

FEAR is NOT an **acceptable excuse!**

We are **100%** responsible for our **choice:**

Controlling

How

Our

Intentions

Create

Experiences

Tool # 5

Feel the fear and do it anyway!

This is the title of another great book,

"Feel the Fear and Do It Anyway" - Dr. Susan Jeffries

It also is a great tool when you put it in to practice!

There are **2** more strategies I'd like to share:

1) Recognize that fear is really our brain *playing a trick* on us! It may help you to look at fear in the following way:

$$\textbf{F}\text{ind}$$

$$\textbf{E}\text{motion}$$

$$\textbf{A}\text{lters}$$

$$\textbf{R}\text{eality}$$

2) This next strategy is another one I learned from a Jack Canfield training:

You can do this either standing or sitting.

Pinch your thumb and 1st or 2nd finger together on both hands.

Hold them out in front and to the sides of you.

Now repeat this mantra in a low 'hum':

"Oh what the heck,
go for it anyways"

(If you don't want to make a scene, you can always say it in your head!)

I love this strategy!!!!! One of my favorites!

It's a great way to break through the old fear recording that plays in our head!

I think it works so great because it combines **the mind & the body**...

Why Wellness?

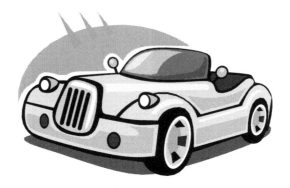

HOW MANY CARS HAVE YOU OWNED?

or

HOW MANY HAVE BEEN IN YOUR HOUSEHOLD?

(This includes new & used ones!)

1

3

5

Maybe More!

(Depending on your age of course!)

Imagine….

You had 1 car that had to last you a lifetime.

How well would you take care of that car?!

If you are like most people,

you would probably take very good care of it,

including regular *preventive* maintenance!

Well, I love to be the one to break the news to you…

We **ONLY** get one vehicle to *live our life with!*

ONE BODY that has to
LAST A LIFETIME!

What is Wellness?

For many years, I used to define wellness as

"optimal health".

I liked the definition because <u>not</u> <u>everyone's</u> the same.

The person who has asthma will be different
from the person who does not,
yet they can still strive for wellness.

A couple years ago, as I was preparing to deliver a
keynote speech in North Carolina, I came across an
even better definition. I use this one now, exclusively.

The National Wellness Institute's:

**"Wellness is an active process of becoming
aware of and making choices towards a more
successful existence."**

After all, **wellness is the key** to having

this **one body be able to last us a lifetime!**

Is It Hunger, Stress, Or Loneliness?

Substitution

I believe this area gets paid the *least amount* of attention in the discussion on quitting.

As I just explained - for many, smoking may be their *GO-TO* TOOL….making it a survival tool!

Cigarettes are like a smoker's 'Swiss army knife!'

They *USE* them to 'fix' problems

in *a lot of different areas of life*:

Work…**Family**… **Relationships**… **School**…

When people ⊘ , they can easily substitute another **Survival Tool** in place of cigarettes. This is called "substitution"!

The **#1** substitution is FOOD!

The next chapters will help you WIN this BATTLE!

When it comes to hunger, there are two types!

We must start to pay attention & become aware of which one it is that has us eating!

Hunger

Emotional	**Physical**
Comes on **suddenly**	Is **gradual**
Felt **above** the neck (craving for ice cream)	Felt **below** the neck (growling stomach)
Must be **Certain** Food (like pizza or chocolate)	**Any** food will do (just needs fuel!)
Wants to be satisfied **instantly**	**Can wait**
Guilt	**No** guilt

Source: Researchers from University of Texas
Counseling & Mental Health Center

Carol's 2 Steps to Success

1) *Identify the Source*

Is it physical hunger?

or

Is it emotional hunger?

2) *Take Action!*

If it's physical hunger –

FEED it with healthy choices

If it's emotional hunger –

FEEL IT

&

RELEASE IT!

Creating the
Release Valves

All Shook Up

Has this ever happened to you?

You go into a store & buy either a liter of

diet coke or some raspberry seltzer.

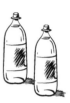

Along the way, you are very careful not to shake it up!

Then one evening that next week,

you go to pour yourself a glass,

your mind busy paying attention to dinner on the stove

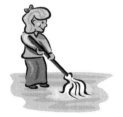

and ....

SPLASH.......

stuff comes flying out of the bottle you just opened -

all over you & the floor creating a mess!

Sometimes in life,

it doesn't matter how careful we are.

Things will still get shaken up!

I believe the same thing happens

when it comes to our emotions!

Sometimes **WE** get *shaken up!*

And if we aren't careful,

we end up with a **BIG EMOTIONAL MESS!**

If you're to have any success at moving away from

using cigarettes as a way of coping with your emotions,

then

you've got to learn a little more about

managing them in a healthy way!

I want to introduce you to my system I call

"The Feeling's Pendulum".

Take a look at the next page
& see where you would put yourself!

The Feelings Pendulum

What Do You Do
With Your Feelings?

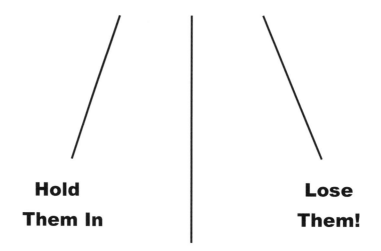

**Hold
Them In**

**Manage
Them**

**Lose
Them!**

So which one did you pick?

If you are a "Manage Them", congratulations!

You obviously know what to do with your emotions!

If you are a "Hold Them In",

I am going to guess at times, you also can "Lose It"!

Finally, if you start at "Lose Them", & stay at

"Lose Them", **don't worry**! Help is on the way!

PS. "Lose Them" has 2 directions to it –
OUTWARD – comes out on & affects *others*
INWARD – Stays in & affects only *YOU*
(Called **RELAPSE**)

I like using a pendulum because it
perfectly illustrates just how difficult can be to

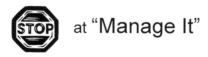 at "Manage It"

if you start up on either end.

Momentum makes it difficult to stop!

I have another way I like to teach people to

think about emotions and how to manage them!

First, let me ask:

"Have you ever said something
 you wished had *never*

come out of your mouth?"

I think most people can relate to experiences like this!!!

Here's **why it happens –**

When our emotions are so high that their level
is up to our nose – simply by opening our mouth
to speak they will come SPILLING OUT!

When things are at this high of a level –
we will have **NO CONTROL** over what comes out!

Best not to say anything when emotions are this high!
WAIT! There's an even worse level to be at....

BRAIN LEVEL!

When we are filled with emotion up above our 's

we *lose control over our brain!*

It's like our brain gets **"flooded"** & we can end up

DOING STUPID THINGS,

not just saying them!

[Okay, maybe this hasn't happened to you. But I am

sure you can think of other people this might describe!]

Managing emotions requires a process

which has us do two things:

1) **STOP** the level from rising any higher.

2) **RELEASE SOME** so that the level will drop.

IMPORTANT:

It is only when the level is *lower* than the neck,

that we should attempt to talk!

If our emotion is right at neck level it'll *still* **CHOKE US!**

STOP the Level From Rising!

There are many ways to **STOP** our level of emotions from rising. Remember, there are both healthy AND unhealthy ways!

Think of **SURVIVAL TOOLS** vs. **LIFETOOLS!**

Some of the **unhealthy** ways: (SURVIVAL TOOLS)

Smoke   Eat   Drink   Shut down   Isolate

Avoidance   ***Smoke more***   Ignore things

Sleep   Use negative self talk   **SMOKE!**

Some of the ***healthy*** ways: (LIFETOOLS)

Take a time out   Belly Breathing   Count to 10

Set limits   Decline to talk about it anymore

Guided Imagery   Consider the Source   Listen to music

Use the Serenity Prayer   Walk Away

Focus on something else   Use ✚ self talk

Change your thought pattern   meditation   prayer

'It is what it is'   All passive relaxation techniques

Decline the invitation to fight   walk outside & look UP!

RELEASE So the Level Will Drop

In order to **release emotion**……

muscle involvement is required.

Think of it like we are bailing water out of a boat.

We must take ACTION

in order to get the water out!

The same principle applies to emotions.

We must take ACTION to get the emotion out!

It requires we involve 'muscles'

to actually **create the release**!

The quick **3** I throw out are easy to remember:

Walk   Talk   Write!

If you remember nothing more than these & put them in to practice, you will be on your way to *managing your emotions rather than having them manage you!*

PS. You will also discover many more active releases

in the next chapter on stress!

After all, emotions can often be *our response to stress!*

In my workshops, I will take a couple liter bottles

 & hand them out to different people to

shake them up really good.

I want to use them to reinforce a point

about managing emotions.......

Our **emotions** are just like the pressure that builds up

inside those bottles when they get **" ALL SHOOK UP!"**

It doesn't do any good to simply **STOP** the shaking!!!!!

We must also create the release!!!

Think about it for a moment.

What happens if someone takes a bottle that's

been **"ALL SHOOK UP!"** & sets it

back in the refrigerator or in the cupboard?

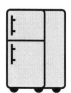

The pressure doesn't go anywhere!!!!!

UNTIL….

it just ends up dumping a mess on
the next unsuspecting person!

The same happens with our emotions….

We end up **dumping them out on the next person**!

To prevent this from happening we

MUST USE A RELEASE!

(Kind of like when you take a bottle and twist the cap a
little bit at a time to let some of the pressure out!)

There is another **IMPORTANT** point to remember….

We can't often tell just by looking at the bottle
whether or not it has any pressure built up inside!

Just as we often can't tell looking at a person
whether or not
have any emotional pressure built up inside!!!

The best strategy is PREVENTION! Approach with
caution & be prepared to move quickly out of the way!

Stress Management
Made Simple!

"Raise your hand if you know STRESS is not good for your health?"

When I ask this question in my workshops – everyone in there will raise their hand! I'm sure you too would also raise your hand! So we can stop here, right?   *WRONG*!

Even though we all *know* **STRESS** is *not good for our health*, very few people do anything about it!

So I like to take a different approach…..

I focus on helping people **DO** something about it!

After all, if we can reduce our **STRESS** levels,
we can actually cut our risk of
dying from heart disease, cancer, & diabetes.
AND AS IMPORTANTLY: Returning to smoking

I want you to get a piece of paper & pen right now,
before you go to the next page.

Don't go there until you have them ready!

97

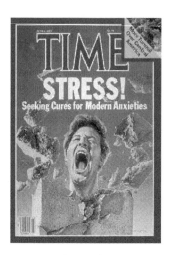

What do you think of when you see this?

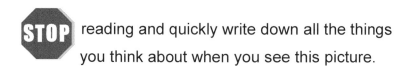 reading and quickly write down all the things you think about when you see this picture.

When you are done writing, let's continue!

I love doing this exercise! What I find is that each person usually has something different come to mind

when they see or hear the word **STRESS**.

When I do this exercise in a workshop, we get a lot of different answers.

I'd like to share some of them with you!

They may be very similar to what you've written down.

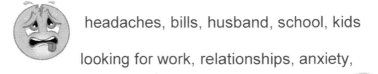 headaches, bills, husband, school, kids

looking for work, relationships, anxiety,

loss of control, can't sleep, shopping,

break up, family, job interviews, money,

birthdays, not working, overwhelmed, life, tuition,

kid's schedules, holidays, Dr.'s appointments, driving

Now here is an important part for you to understand:

What is STRESS?

"A response to a situation or change."

Let's talk about "response" for a moment.

Usually the response is something we don't

have much control over

once it starts.

Kind of like a reflex –
the doctor hits my knee and my leg moves!

Has this ever happened to you?

You have a big event going on in your life.

Let's say an interview for a job.

First off, you don't sleep very well the night before.

Then as you are getting ready,

your stomach starts to twist and turn.

You are about to have a case of the 'runs'!

Now, who would *actually let these responses happen*?

 NO ONE!

This is the thing about STRESS –

Once it hits, we <u>don't</u> <u>get</u> <u>to</u> <u>have</u> too much control!

Before we move on, I also want to point out

something else that is VERY important:

STRESS does not come one size fits all!

Here's what I mean by this:

1st we must realize that **'the change or situation'** does not always come in a negative form!

We can have # POSITIVE

changes or situations that can trigger a response.

Look at your list:

Can you identify some POSITIVE stress sources on it?

If you didn't write any down,

can you think of any right now that you could add?

2nd we must realize **'the change or situation'** does not come in just one size!

It can be either BIG or SMALL.

Think about it for a moment…..

What happens to your stress level when the kids are

running 5 minutes late in the morning?

or

You are running 5 minutes late for an appointment?

3rd
we must realize **'the change or situation'**
may be stressful for one person but *not another*!

STRESS is a very personal thing!

Just because something may not be *STRESS to me*
does not mean it *may not be STRESS to you!*

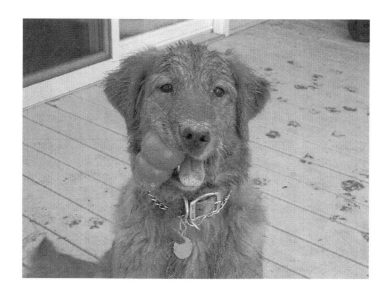

I wanted to share with you one of my
POSITIVE STRESSES!

Now that we have a little clearer picture of STRESS

LET"S DO SOMETHING ABOUT IT!!

Do you have kids?

Has your washer ever been broken?

Do you hate to do laundry?

If you answered YES to any of the above,
then you already may be a bit of a
stress expert & not even know it!

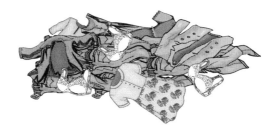

This is the pile of laundry after just 1 week!
(And you have NO ONE to do it for you!)

Heading in to the next week, things are so busy

that you don't have any time to do laundry.

It has to **wait** until next weekend.

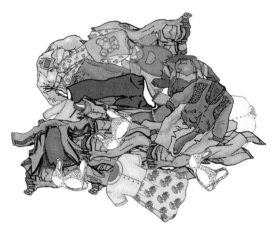

This is the pile of laundry you are looking at week 2!

It starts to GROW BIGGER!!

But wait…..

There just isn't enough time to get it all done.

You've got an evening function this week,

it's your neighbor's birthday, and

you still have to go shopping for a present.

Everyone has enough clothes to last them

one more week…..

Besides, there isn't anything happening next weekend.

So......laundry is put off for another week!

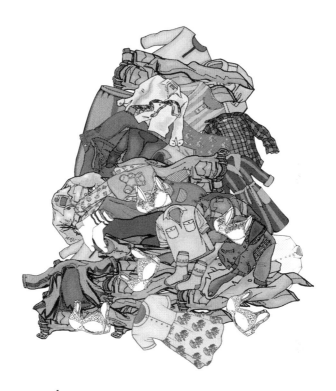

Imagine **how** you would **feel** if you had to look

at a pile of laundry as tall as you?!

What can we do to *keep laundry from piling up*?

Do a load as frequently as possible!

Sometimes we may need to do **2 loads or more** a day!

STRESS is just like laundry!

It piles up!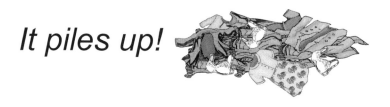

Sure!

You can *pretend* it's not there!

Maybe even try to hide it!

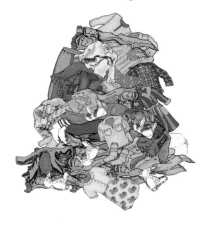

Whether you see it or not –

it still keeps *piling up*!

Solution # 1:

Do **at least** one load a day of

Stress Laundry!

[This *means you must select and do at least one of the activities listed in the following pages. Don't rely on the same one or two. Try things you've never done before!*]

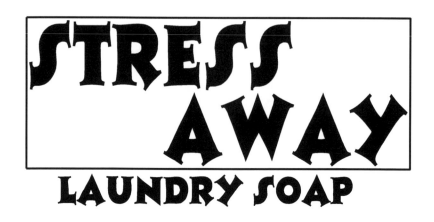

LAUNDRY SOAP

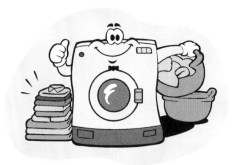

Guaranteed to lighten any day!

Directions:

* Use at least one time daily.

* Separate in to piles if
    too large for one load.

* May need to do multiple loads!

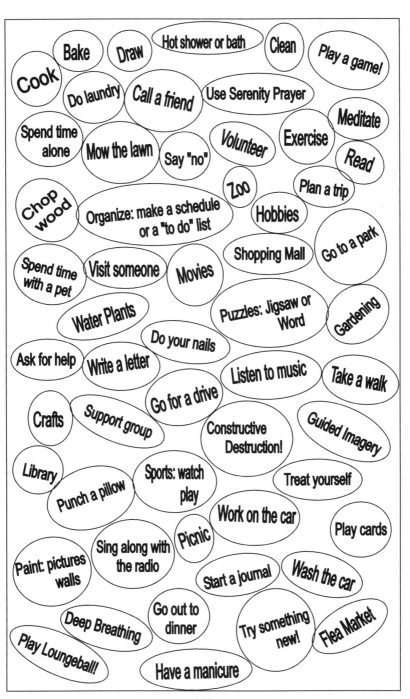

Cook
Bake
Draw
Hot shower or bath
Clean
Play a game!
Do laundry
Call a friend
Use Serenity Prayer
Meditate
Spend time alone
Mow the lawn
Say "no"
Volunteer
Exercise
Read
Chop wood
Organize: make a schedule or a "to do" list
Zoo
Plan a trip
Hobbies
Go to a park
Spend time with a pet
Visit someone
Movies
Shopping Mall
Water Plants
Puzzles: Jigsaw or Word
Gardening
Do your nails
Ask for help
Write a letter
Listen to music
Take a walk
Go for a drive
Crafts
Support group
Constructive Destruction!
Guided Imagery
Library
Punch a pillow
Sports: watch play
Treat yourself
Work on the car
Play cards
Picnic
Sing along with the radio
Paint: pictures walls
Start a journal
Wash the car
Go out to dinner
Deep Breathing
Try something new!
Flea Market
Play Loungeball!
Have a manicure

Solution # 2:

Avoid adding to the PILE!

Take steps to **AVOID** the things that cause you STRESS!

Only when I started doing my own laundry did I come to appreciate why my Mom would get so mad when I would change clothes a bunch!!

As you can see, when it comes to **STRESS**
most people are already experts!
Okay, maybe not the person who
takes everything to the dry cleaners!

It makes sense, doesn't it?

We all have to do

a little stress laundry everyday!

PS. I wanted to share some of the ways **I avoid**
adding to my pile of **STRESS**:

#1) When I have to go some place new for a speech

or an appointment, I'll go find it ahead of time.

If I can't do that,

I make sure to leave myself extra time to find it.

#2) I plan out my meals for the week & **avoid** the

STRESS of coming home from work &

trying to figure out 'what's for dinner?'

#3) At work, I **avoid** the **STRESS** of not getting things

done by making sure I complete what I'm

working on, before I move on to the next!

(This really use to be a **very big STRESS**, as I had this

habit of skipping around to different tasks &

then feeling like I wasn't accomplishing anything!)

#4) I make sure I get my exercise done each **morning**

this way it's done, and I don't have to worry

about still doing it when I get home from work.

However, there are many things we can't control in life.

Times in LIFE when we seem to get **DUMPED ON**.

I refer to this as

"The Dump Truck O'Stress"

Let me illustrate this next!

Dump Truck O'Stress!

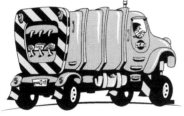

- - - - -

A truck full of 'dirty laundry was
suddenly dropped on your front door...

How would you **FEEL?**　　What would you **DO?**

Here are some pretty natural reactions:

Angry	Give Up
Overwhelmed	Explode
Powerless	Hide
Hopeless	Run

Life's big **STRESS** cause these *same reactions* –

**These are life events & changes that come on
quickly, without warning, and in a big way**

**The equivalent of a dump truck
full of dirty laundry!**

What to do when the Dump Truck O'Stress pulls up:

1. Give yourself permission to **feel the way you do** (Otherwise it just adds to the pile!)

2. Break it in to **smaller piles**
   (Small piles are easier to manage!)

3. Ask for **help** (The more people working on a pile, the better the chance of getting through it!)

4. Make a plan or a **time schedule**
   (This helps keep you focused!)

5. **Prioritize**
   (Figure out what's important to take care of first)

6. Be **realistic**!
   (It may take a while to chip away at the pile)

7. Take it "**one pile at a time**"
   (This makes less stress!)

The Power Tools!

WHETHER YOU THINK YOU CAN

OR

YOU THINK YOU CAN'T...

YOU'RE RIGHT!

HENRY FORD

Brain Power

One of the most powerful tools we have is our brain!

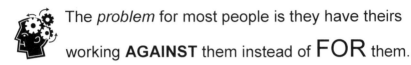 The *problem* for most people is they have theirs working **AGAINST** them instead of FOR them.

The previous quote says it all!
I believe it was written by Henry Ford.
(*I'm not certain as I have heard it many different times!*)

Think about it for a moment……

There are so many great inventors like Henry Ford, the Wright Brothers, & Thomas Edison who **thought they could**, even when *the world thought they couldn't*. In fact, the world believed it impossible!

They learned to harness their brain's power to work FOR THEM allowing their dreams come to life!.

I wonder?

What dreams would you achieve if you believed **YOU COULD!!!!!!**

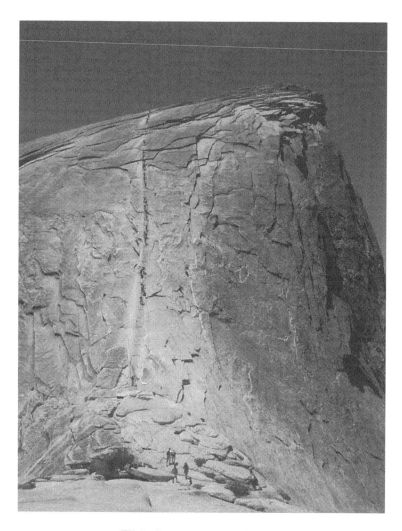

This is my example of:

"If you think you can or you think you can't, You're right"

This is Half Dome, located in *Yosemite National Park*.

This is a view that **most** of the park's
millions of visitors each year will **NEVER** see.....

In order to get where this picture was taken, you have
to hike **8 miles** in to the *back country* of Yosemite.

Of course, it's all up hill! It ends up rising from 4,000
foot elevation in the valley to 8,800 feet at the top.

My brother & I had reached the bottom of the dome.
I can't repeat exactly what he said, but a clean
translation is "Holy Shit!" At that moment our thoughts
of climbing to the top vanished! However, we felt very
proud of our accomplishment just getting to here!

We didn't think we could!

My nieces unexpectedly showed up! We thought they
were ahead of us & half way up the dome by now!
Excited & eager for us to ALL reach the top,
they encouraged us to give it a try. After all,
we had come this far.....

They got us thinking we could!

And we did!

This is the view from the top!

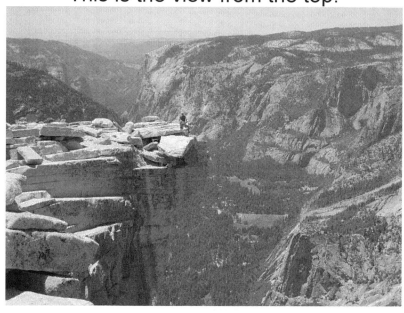

Yosemite Valley is down below!

I don't know who the guy was!
I just thought he was brave.

What are YOU stopping
yourself from doing?!

A Life Changed

It comes as quite a shock to my patients & colleagues
I *was once* the **most negative, pessimistic person!**

I didn't think anything could go my way.

I was working **12** hours a day and

still barely paying my bills.

I made **less** at my job than what I paid to go to college.
For me, there was *nothing good about anything.*

But then in 1989 I had a moment that was life changing.
I will share more about this in a moment. Since then,
I've tried to learn as much as I can about using the
power of thoughts as a tool for transformation &
wellness. My study has impacted both my personal and
professional life. As I learn new ideas & strategies, I try
to incorporate them not only in to my life but also in to
my work with others. After all, what good is knowledge
if it is not shared! I'm on a mission to share
what I have learned with others!

I'm thankful for the opportunity to share it with you.

I had mentioned earlier that I had a moment in 1989
which changed my life around.

It was a blessing hidden in heart ache.

&

has truly shaped the life I live today.

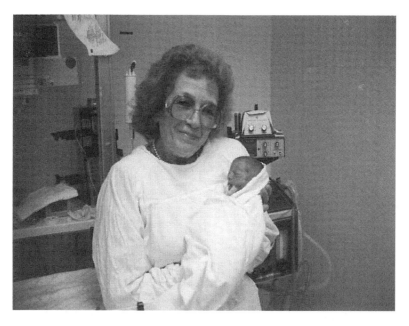

This is a picture of my mother taken December, 1988.
She is holding my nephew, Christopher.

It is my mother who gave me
the greatest gift a person could receive.
Let me explain…..

My mother had called me at work to tell me her doctor wanted her to come in to the hospital right away. It was only when we got in to a room at the emergency room my mother finally told me about the cancer.

It is *no surprise* she had kept this information to herself. After all, she'd done it before.

That afternoon I was on the phone with my sisters out in California making plans to get my mother out West so she could have a chance to see everyone.

Those plans <u>never</u> <u>happened</u>........

My mother ended up passing away that very night. With the tears, sadness, grief and heartache came the greatest gift I could ever receive:

It doesn't matter what we plan for tomorrow ~
We must live our life today as if it were the only one.

We must live One Day At A Time

I like to share the **power of serenity** that goes along with being able to live one day at a time.

I have an exercise I created & I'd like to share with you.

First, read the following:

YESTERDAY, TODAY, and TOMORROW

There are two days in every week that we need not worry about, two days that must be kept free from fear and apprehension.

One is **YESTERDAY**, with it's mistakes & cares, it's faults & blunders, it's aches & pains. Yesterday has passed, forever beyond our control. All the money in the world cannot bring back yesterday. We cannot undo a single   act we performed. Nor can we erase a single word we've said – Yesterday is gone!

The other day we must not worry about is **TOMORROW**, with it's impossible adversaries, it's burden, it's hopeful promise and poor performance. Tomorrow is beyond our control!

Tomorrow's sun will rise either in splendor or behind a mask of clouds – but it will rise. And until it does, we have no stake in tomorrow, for it is yet unborn.

This leaves only one day – **TODAY**. Any person can fight the battles of just one day. It is only when we add the burdens of yesterday & tomorrow that we break down.

It is not the experience of today that drives people mad—it is the remorse of bitterness for something which happened yesterday, and the dread of what tomorrow may bring. LET US LIVE ONE DAY AT A TIME!!!!

(Author Unknown)

Second, take a blank piece of paper and
write Yesterday, Tomorrow, & Today on it
so it looks like this:

```
┌─────────────────────────────────┐
│                                 │
│           Yesterday             │
│                                 │
│                                 │
│                                 │
│           Tomorrow              │
│                                 │
│                                 │
│                                 │
│            Today                │
│                                 │
│                                 │
│                                 │
└─────────────────────────────────┘
```

Under "Yesterday" -

I want you to write down all the things from **the past**
(from yesterday or 20 years ago) that still occupy your
thoughts. This includes regrets, resentments, hurts,
the I shoulda-woulda-coulda's, guilt's, & anything else!

Under Tomorrow -

I want you to write down all the things from **the future** that occupy your thoughts. This includes worries, fears, "what-if's", uncertainties, hopes, & dreams!

Under TODAY -

I want you to look back over the things you've written under yesterday & tomorrow. Ask yourself this **?** about *each* of the items you have listed:

"Is there anything I can **DO** about that TODAY?"

If there is, write down under **TODAY** the **SPECIFIC ACTION** you can take.

It must be something you can DO!

If there isn't,
don't write anything under TODAY

Once you have completed this,
there is one last step to take!

Fold the paper *just above* where **TODAY** is written.

Now, keep folding it back & forth several times on that same crease. You can even lick it if you want but don't get a paper cut!

Now carefully tear the paper along the crease.

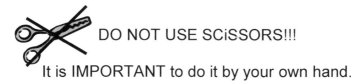 DO NOT USE SCiSSORS!!!
It is IMPORTANT to do it by your own hand.

You should end up with 2 pieces of paper in your hands.

One piece has <u>Yesterday</u> & <u>Tomorrow</u> on it.

Feel free to burn this, rip it up, shred it, and destroy it!

The other piece has TODAY on it.

Hold onto this!

It is the only day we CAN do anything about.

You may need to do repeat this every day until you're able to focus on TODAY!

Another way of looking at it:

'WHY's'

GET US LOST IN THE PAST

'WHAT-IF's'

GET US LOST IN THE FUTURE

CAROL L RICKARD

Are these words you often speak?

If so, they will prevent you from

Living in Today!

One More Power Tool

Another *powerful* **LIFETOOL** for me has long been the Serenity Prayer. I started putting it in to practice in my life after I started working an addictions treatment unit.

I had heard of & was familiar with it; however it wasn't until I was around people who could teach me how to USE IT, that it became one of my primary tools. Just like 'One Day at a Time' - this **LIFETOOL** holds

The Power of Peace & Serenity

My strongest test of this tool came in the summer of 2006. It was in July when my sister Kris suddenly died.

Since I live in central New Jersey, I flew out of Philadelphia. My flight got out of the gate right on time....but once on the way to the runway; we sat there for almost **2** hours.

I was to catch a connecting flight out of Salt Lake City in to Reno. My brother & his family, flying from

Virginia, were on the same flight out of Salt Lake City. Needless to say – I never caught up with them.

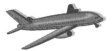

My delay in Philly had me miss the connecting flight. The worst news came when I was booked on a flight the next morning: **1 hour** after the funeral was to start. Now here I was stranded the night in Salt Lake City.

Really, what could I do? So, I kept the Serenity Prayer repeating in my head over & over & over again.

I called my family from the airport in Salt Lake City & informed them I wouldn't even be leaving Salt Lake City **until the next day and AFTER the funeral had already started.**

As I kept repeating the Serenity Prayer, I let the tears flow. I had a lot of mixed emotions and I knew it wasn't a good idea to hold them in.

In the past, under stressful conditions like these I would have had a major migraine before the plane ever landed in Utah.

Turns out, I didn't get a migraine all weekend.
This was despite not getting to my sister's house
until AFTER all the days events had taken place.
My **LIFETOOL** held me steady!

As I said a little earlier in this book, there are many
times in life we don't get to choose what happens.....

We *DO* get to *CHOOSE* our *RESPONSE* to them!

God grant me,

The *Serenity* to accept the things
I cannot change

The *Courage* to change the things I can

And the *Wisdom* to know the difference

Here is my shortened version of it:

Can I do anything about it right now?

If not, I just have to **let it go!**

Important:

I would like to make this point about *'Letting Go'* or
as they say in recovery circles: *'Let go and let God'*

We cannot let go of something
we have not allowed
ourselves to feel!

In order to 'let go' of something –

we must first **FEEL the FEELINGS** connected to it

and then

'Let Go'!

(One way to think of this is we simply have something
come in through one ear, acknowledge it (feel it!),
and move on out through the other side!)

Another way I explain 'Let Go' to my patients:

Leave

Everything

To

Gods

Ownership

And one last way to practice "Letting Go"!

Write down what it is you are trying to
'let go' of on a small slip of paper.

Then do one of the following with the slip:

✴ Put it in a special box you have decorated

(Many people refer to these as a God Box
or a Worry Box. You can find all types of
boxes at your local craft store)

✴ Put it in a special book

(This could be a book of worship or
another special book of yours)

✴ Throw it in a fireplace

(If you don't have one, it could be any other
safe way to destroy it by burning!)

✴ Shred it up

(This could be as simple as throwing
it in the shredder or tearing it by hand
in to a bunch of little itty, bitty pieces!

You will notice the one thing these all have in common

is they **REQUIRE ACTION BE TAKEN!**

Instead of just trying to do this '*all in our head*',

we get our entire body involved in the process!

I believe it is this **PRINCIPLE OF DOING**

which leads us to great success.

When our mind starts to go back

to thinking about it again.....

Be prepared that it will!

Our mind <u>will</u> try to hold on to things!!

We can also remind ourselves we have "gotten rid"

of **what** it is trying to access again!

A couple more WordTools!

Find

An

Important

Lesson

Using

Real

Experiences!

The

Recognizable

Incident

Generating

Great

Emotional

Response

Giving

Respect

And

Thanks

Everyday

For

Unbelievable

Life

Wrapping Things Up

We started off by taking a look at

WHY it can be so hard to quit smoking.

If you try to take on the challenge to

all on your own, you are waging a fight against

BIOLOGY.

There is a high probability you'll …. **LOSE!**

There are so many proven ways & resources

to increase your odds of success.

Please use them!!!

NRT, Counseling, Quit Lines, Support!

Next we looked at **HOW** you may be using your

cigarettes as a 'Swiss army knife'!

My hope is that you now have *enough*

of the healthier tools to be able to retire

the 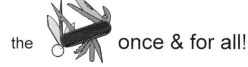 once & for all!

Even if you're able to use many of these new tools,

It is VERY IMPORTANT

you keep in mind tobacco use & dependence is

a chronic disease process.

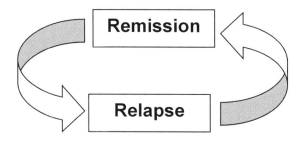

Relapse can be a great opportunity to learn

what you may need to adjust to go back & again:

KICK Cigarettes Butts!

Remember, learning anything new requires

practice for it to become a new habit.

Change is a process!!

Do not get discouraged should you find yourself

slipping back to old behaviors every now & then.

Learn from the 'slips' and move on.

Two steps forward, one step back

still has us *moving closer* to our goals.

Try this exercise!

Start on one side of a room.

Take two steps forward & one step back.

Now, do it again!

Two steps forward & one step back.

Repeat this process *at least* 2 more times!

Are you closer to the other side

of the room than where you started?

YES!!!

So when your brain starts to yell at you:

'you're going backwards' Yell back! "No I'm not!!"

We then looked at the issue

of *SUBSTITUTION:*

The goal here is you start becoming aware of

WHY

you are putting that food in your mouth!

Is it *physical* hunger or *emotional* hunger?

Step 1 - Use the guidelines we talked
about to help you figure this out.

Step 2 - You must do one of the following:

FEED physical hunger something healthy!

Or

FEEL the emotions & then release them.

Again, since this is new,
it may take some practice for you to get better at it!!

Don't beat yourself up if you stumble.

We then focused on:

STRESS. MANAGEMENT MADE SIMPLE!

The goal here is to have gotten you thinking differently about STRESS & seeing how easy it is to do something about it!

Remember, the best way to **stress less** is

DO A LOAD OF STRESS LAUNDRY EVERDAY!

As you become more aware of when it is

PILING UP,

You may need to do extra loads!

And of course, the BEST strategy is to

avoid adding to the pile in the first place.

Be on the look out:

STRESS comes in all shapes & sizes!

The last area we focused on: **THE POWER TOOLS**.

Once you can get your brain working

for you rather than against you –

YOU CAN ACCOMPLISH ANYTHING!

Our thoughts & the words we choose to use

are the paint brushes we use to create our life!

If you take nothing else away from this chapter

I can only hope that it is how to use

One Day at A Time

&

The Serenity Prayer

The Key!

1) False – Nicotine causes addiction, not cancer

2) False – You can!

3) True – 50% is correct

4) False – No tobacco is safe!

5) False – Not yet!

6) False – 90%

7) False - 65

8) True – Combo can increase success!

9) True – Only 4-7% quit cold turkey!

10) False – It only takes 10 seconds!

Additional Resources

www.BecomeAnEx.org

www.QuitSolutions.org

www.SmokeFree.Gov

www.cdc.gov/tips

www.lung.org

www.quitnet.com

www.cancer.org

References

- Centers for Disease Control and Prevention. **Best Practices for Comprehensive Tobacco Control Programs — 2014.**Atlanta: U.S. Department of Health and Human Services, Centers for Disease Control and Prevention, National Center for Chronic Disease Prevention and Health Promotion, Office on Smoking and Health, 2014.

- U.S. Department of Health and Human Services. *The Health Consequences of Smoking—50 Years of Progress. A Report of the Surgeon General.* Atlanta, GA: U.S. Department of Health and Human Services, Centers for Disease Control and Prevention, National Center for Chronic Disease Prevention and Health Promotion, Office on Smoking and Health, 2014. Printed with corrections, January 2014.

- US Food and Drug Administration's Center for Tobacco for Tobacco Products Website

- Tobacco Dependence Treatment Specialist Training Manual. University of Medicine and Dentistry of New Jersey. Tobacco Dependence Program. 1/2011

About the Author

Carol Rickard, LCSW, TTS has written over a dozen publications & conducted national training workshops on stress and wellness. She is the founder and CEO of Well YOUniversity, LLC, a global leader in health education & training, whose mission is to empower individuals with the tools and supports to achieve lifelong wellness.

Carol is a popular speaker / trainer at all types of conferences and events. She provides community education for hospitals, continuing education programs, staff professional development and CEU/CME courses. Her high energy, unique approach and compelling presentation change thinking and inspire participants to take action towards L.I.F.E wellness (**L**iving **I**ntentionally & **F**ully **E**ngaged).

Carol can be reached at Carol@WellYOUniversity.com.

Facebook: www.FaceBook.com/WellYOUniversity

Want to Insure Your Success?

Master the Tools Even Faster With This One of a Kind Program.

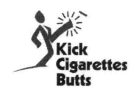 **Kick Cigarettes Butts**

The Ultimate 4-Step Success System

Kick Cigarettes Butts home video program provides you with some additional training to **master the tools** needed to help *ensure* you'll be successful in quitting tobacco!

This 4 DVD set includes:

# 1 – KCB Success Blueprint	(Value: $227)
# 2 – The Feelings Pendulum	(Value: $227)
# 3 – Stress Away	(Value: $227)
# 4 – The Anger Umbrella	(Value: $227)

Total Value: $ 908

For a *Limited Time Only* $197.00 at:

www.KickCigarettesButts.com

Please visit us at:

www.WellYOUniversity.com

Sign up for weekly motivational e-quote!

Check out our upcoming FREE webinars!

Learn more about our training programs.

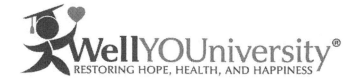

Email us your success story at:

Success@WellYOUniversity.com

Register This Book and Get Free Updates and Free Videos

To get free updates to this book and access to videos that will show you how to utilize strategies in this book and an invitation to online interactive livecasts to meet the author & ask questions, visit www.TheBenefitsOfSmokingBonus.com or text BOS to 58885 or text your name and email address to (609) 455-1224 Or scan this QR code:

35269329R00090

Made in the USA
Charleston, SC
02 November 2014